Obachola Julien ADETOKOUN
Sié Hermann POODA
Ernest Wendemanegde SALOU

Biological control of tsetse flies, vectors of trypanosomes.

Obachola Julien ADETOKOUN
Sié Hermann POODA
Ernest Wendemanegde SALOU

Biological control of tsetse flies, vectors of trypanosomes.

Evaluation of the insecticidal properties of essential oils against tsetse flies, vectors of animal trypanosomes.

ScienciaScripts

Cover image: www.ingimage.com

This book is a translation from the original published under ISBN 978-613-9-50444-2.

Publisher:
Sciencia Scripts
is a trademark of
Dodo Books Indian Ocean Ltd. and OmniScriptum S.R.L publishing group

120 High Road, East Finchley, London, N2 9ED, United Kingdom
Str. Armeneasca 28/1, office 1, Chisinau MD-2012, Republic of Moldova, Europe
Managing Directors: Ieva Konstantinova, Victoria Ursu
info@omniscriptum.com

Printed at: see last page
ISBN: 978-620-8-53307-6

TABLE OF CONTENTS

DEDICATION

*To my mother **BABATOUNDE Charlotte**, this iron lady, this Amazon, who has always believed in me. Thank you so much for your unconditional love and your prayers. You are an inexhaustible source of motivation. I won't let you down. I love you all.*

*To my father **ADETOKOUN Emmanuel**, You fought until the end. Thank you for your advice and encouragement.*

*To my **brothers and sisters** Fabrice, Bienvenu, Bernadette, Sabine, Marceline, Nathalie and Noélie. You are an inexhaustible source of motivation. I won't let you down. You are the best brothers and sisters in the world.*

ACKNOWLEDGEMENTS

I would like to express my gratitude and appreciation to :

- ***Professor Hassan Bismarck NACRO,*** *President of Nazi Boni University, thank you so much for welcoming us to your University;*
- ***Professor Abdoulaye DIABATE****, Director of Research at IRSS/Bobo-Dioulasso, Director of CEA/ITECH-MTV. You are more than a role model for the students and a reference in the world of medical entomology. Thank you for the trust you place in your students and thank you so much for welcoming us;*
- ***Dr Guiguigbaza-Kossigan DAYO****, Senior Researcher, Director General of the International Centre for Research and Development on Livestock in Subhumid Zones (CIRDES), thank you so much for welcoming us to your research centre;*
- ***Dr Dari Yannick Frédéric Da****, Senior Researcher at IRSS-DRO, Deputy Coordinator of research activities at CEA/ITECH-MTV. Thank you for your support, advice and guidance;*
- ***Dr Moussa NAMOUNTOUGOU****, senior lecturer at Nazi Boni University, deputy coordinator of CEA/ITECH-MTV's academic activities. Thank you for your support, advice and guidance;*
- ***Dr Michel GOMGNIMBOU****, Associate Professor of Molecular Biology at Nazi Boni University and supervisor of this dissertation. Thank you for sharing your time, experience and skills with us. We were fortunate to benefit from your teaching;*
- ***Dr Sié Hermann POODA****, Senior Lecturer at the University of Dédougou, researcher in the Vector-borne Diseases and Biodiversity Unit (UMAVeB) of CIRDES, for having agreed to co-direct my training course and for having made himself available for the completion of this work. Thank you for sharing your time, experience and skills with me and for the effort you made to improve the quality of the writing of this thesis. I have learned a great deal from you. This work is a good example of what you have taught me. Many thanks for the success of this work;*
- ***Dr Abel BIGUEZOTON****, Research Fellow at CIRDES, Head of the Vector-borne Diseases and Biodiversity Unit (UMAVeB) at CIRDES, thank you very much for welcoming us to your Unit. Thank you for your advice and guidance;*

- ***Dr Ernest SALOU****, Senior Lecturer at Nazi Boni University, head of the entomology and vector control team in the Vector-borne Diseases and Biodiversity Unit (UMAVeB) at CIRDES. Thank you for sharing your time, experience and skills with us. We were fortunate to benefit from your teaching;*
- ***Dr Soudah BOMA****, Research Fellow at CIRDES, member of the entomology and vector control team of the Vector-borne Diseases and Biodiversity Unit (UMAVeB) at CIRDES. Thank you for sharing your time, experience and skills with us;*
- ***Dr Prudenciène A. AGBOHO****, Research Associate at CIRDES, member of the entomology (tsetse fly) and vector control team of the Vector-borne Diseases and Biodiversity Unit (UMAVeB) at CIRDES. Thank you for sharing your time, experience and skills with us;*
- ***Dr Razaki OSSE****, lecturer and researcher at the National University Agriculture in the Republic of Korea Benin for your assistance throughout my training;*
- *The CIRDES **technicians**, in particular Wilfrid YONI, Lassina SANOGO, Céné BILA and Issiaka BARRY, for helping me to complete my work;*
- *my **fellow trainees** at CIRDES, in particular Armand LALEYE, Kassamba KOROTIMI and Liliane OUEDRAOGO;*
- *all **the CIRDES staff** for good working atmosphere in I carried out my work my work ;*
- *all the **students in my year**, especially Armand LALEYE, Issac OUMAR, José N'TSOUKPOE, Sylvie YERBANGA and Gladys SANOU. I had a great time and learned a lot from you. We will always be a family;*
- *the **teaching staff and management team at CEA/ITECH-MTV** for the richness and quality of their teaching and the efforts they have made to provide students with a high-quality education;*
- *My **colleagues** Bonnet vert in Bobo-Dioulasso **and** Kossam Lobam in Ouagadougou for your assistance and invaluable advice;*
- *to the **members of the Jury** for having accepted, in spite of your duties, to judge the quality of this work. Your observations and criticisms will be invaluable in improving this work. It is a great honour for you to contribute your advice and recommendations to the perfection of this work.*
- *all those who, one way or another, contributed to the production of this work.*

SUMMARY

The tsetse fly, a major vector in transmission of trypanosomes to animals and humans, is a constraint on the development of agriculture and livestock farming in Africa. In order to overcome this constraint, conventional activities to suppress tsetse populations are proving costly for poor rural communities. In addition, the uncontrolled use of chemical insecticides is causing environmental problems. Simple, inexpensive and environmentally friendly control methods therefore need to be identified. With the aim of finding alternatives to synthetic chemical insecticides for the control of tsetse fly vectors of animal trypanosomes, we evaluated the insecticidal potential of essential oils by topical application to the dorsal surface of the thorax and by forced tarsal contact on 1-day-old males of all genera of Glossina palpalis gambiensis at the Centre International de Recherche - Développement sur l'Elevage en zone Subhumide (CIRDES). A study of the insecticidal properties of the essential oils showed that they were effective against Glossina palpalis gambiensis. A dose of 1µl of all the essential oils applied topically to 1-day-old males of Glossina palpalis gambiensis, all generals, resulted in 100% mortality after 24 hours. The results of this study showed that these essential oils have interesting insecticidal properties against Glossina palpalis gambiensis and could be used as an alternative to synthetic chemical insecticides.

Key words : Glossina palpalis gambiensis, Animal trypanosome, Essential oils, CIRDES.

INTRODUCTION

Haematophagous insects, particularly tsetse flies, stomoxes and tabanids, a threat to the development of livestock farming in sub-Saharan Africa (Bouyer, F. E. 2015). The harmful effects of these insects can be seen in the blood loss of livestock and the transmission of pathogens that cause viral, bacterial or parasitic diseases. African animal trypanosomiasis is a parasitic disease caused by parasites of the genus Trypanosoma, transmitted by the tsetse fly (biological vector) and also by mechanical vectors such as tabanids and stomoxes (Solano et al., 2010). The prevalence of African animal trypanosomiasis remains high in most of sub-Saharan Africa, where it is considered to be the most important vector-borne disease with a major impact on nutritional security (Simo et al., 2015). It causes economic losses totalling 4.75 billion dollars a year (Swallow, 2000). Vector control has traditionally been achieved through the application of chemical insecticides, based mainly on the use of conventional insecticides such as organophosphates and pyrethroids (Zahran et al., 2017) on livestock, by spraying and bathing (Bauer et al., 1995; Gimonneau et al., 2016; Vale et al., 2015). However, their massive and continuous use has led to various drawbacks, such as side effects on non-target organisms and the environment, with the risk of contamination or accumulation in the soil, water and harvested produce. All this has led to the development of resistance in non-target insects and health risks for users (Carlos, 2010). The use of plant extracts as insecticides has been known for a long time. They are the best alternatives because they have less impact on the environment (Gitaari et al., 2018). To offset the massive and uncontrolled use of chemical insecticides, it seems sensible to find alternative methods that take environmental requirements into account. Nowadays, the use of plant compounds with insecticidal and repellent properties is enjoying a revival in vector control (Akono et al., 2012). The repellent and insecticidal potential of essential oils has shown encouraging results against cotton pests, Cymbopogon schoenanthus (Bokobana et al., 2014), Dysdercus voelkeri schmidt (Nadio et al., 2015); maize pests, Sitophilus zeamais Motsch and Rhyzopertha dominica (Ouedraogo et al., 2016; Felicia et al, 2018); vectors of Plasmodium, Anopheles funestus (Akono et al., 2012), larvae of Anopheles gambiae s. l. (Nkouandou et al, 2020), mosquitoes in tropical areas (Abagli and Alavo, 2020); animal disease vectors, Stomoxys calcitrans (Bastien,2008 ; Savadogo et al,2016) ; Glossina palpalis gambiensis (Bass et al.,2016 ; Yerbanga et al.,2016). However, to our knowledge, there are no published reports on the insecticidal effect of essential oils in Burkina Faso against tsetse flies.The present study was therefore initiated to examine the efficacy of essential oils from six (6) local plants, Cymbopogon citratus, Eucalyptus camaldulensis, Aloysia citriodora, Hyptis suaveolens, Lantana camara, Mentha piperita and combinations of oils from four plants, Cymbopogon citratus , Aloysia citriodora, Lantana camara and Mentha piperita (Ac/Lc formulation, Cc/Mp formulation, Ac/Cc formulation) for the protection of livestock against tsetse flies, the vectors responsible for animal trypanosomoses. This report, which summarises our work, is divided into two parts. The first part is devoted to a literature review on tsetse flies and general information essential oils. The second part presents the materials and methods, the results obtained and the discussion.

PART I
GENERAL INFORMATION AND REVIEW OF LITERATURE

1 General information on tsetse fly

1.1 Systematics of glossins.

Tsetse flies are haematophagous insects belonging to the suborder Brachyceres, the infraorder Cyclorrhaphes, the family Glossinidae and the genus Glossina. According to the general rule of systematics, tsetse flies are classified as follows:

Kingdom Animal

Phylum Arthropods

Class Insects

Order Diptera

Suborder Brachycera

Family Glossinidae

Genus Glossina

Within the genus Glossina, three groups or sub-genera have been distinguished (Hoare, 1972):

- The Austenina subgenus or fusca group (thirteen species and four subspecies), almost all of which are found in the rainforests or in the wide, dense forest galleries of Equatorial Africa;

Species Subspecies

G. fusca G. fusca congolensis

G. fusca fusca

G. nigrofusca G. nigrofusca hopkinsi

G. nigrofusca nigrofusca

G. brevipalpis

G. frezili

G. fuscipleuris

G. haningtoni

G. longipennis

G. medicorum

G. nashi

G. schwetzi

G. severini

G. tabaniformis

G. vanhoofi

- The **sub-genus Nemorhina** (Robineau-Desvoidy, 1830) or "palpalis group" (five species and seven subspecies) which are generally ripariantound mainly in dense vegetation bordering watercourses or living in peri-domestic groves in Central and West Africa;

Species Subspecies
Glossina palpalis
Glossina palpalis gambiensis
Glossina palpalis palpalis
Glossina fuscipes
Glossina fuscipes fuscipes
Glossina fuscipes martinii
Glossina fuscipes quanzensis
Glossina palliicera
Glossina pallicera pallicera
Glossina pallicera newsteadi
Glossina tachinoides Glossina caliginea

- The **subgenus Glossina s. str.** (Zumpt, 1935) or "morsitans group" (five species and three subspecies) found in wooded savannahs and dense thickets, mainly in areas with abundant livestock or wildlife, and distributed throughout the African continent.

Species Subspecies

Glossina morsitans

Glossina morsitans morsitans

Glossina morsitans centralis

Glossina morsitans submorsitans
Glossina austeni
Glossina pallidipes

Glossina longipalpis
Glossina swynnertoni
Of the tsetse species mentioned above, **Glossina palpalis gambiensis,** belonging to the Palpalis group, is the subject of our study.

1.2 Morphology of tsetse fly

Morphologically, tsetse flies are elongated, robust, blackish-brown in colour and can be recognised by the axe-shaped medico-discal cell on the wings. Both sexes are haematophagous and the female lays the pupae, which is a biological characteristic of tsetse flies. The tsetse is always brown or grey-brown in colour, sometimes with a hint of pink or russet red. The body generally has light and dark spots, making the insect difficult to distinguish when it is resting on the bark of a tree, a rock or on the ground. At rest, the tsetse fly normally looks quite slender because its wings are folded over each other instead of spreading outwards at an angle to the body, as is the case with houseflies and most calliphorines. Immediately after a blood meal, the abdomen of the tsetse fly is swollen, rounded and red. Males are generally smaller than females. The abdomen generally has dark spots on a light yellowish background. The tarsi of the hind legs have only the last two segments covered in black hairs (known as "socks"). The male genitalia have upper forfipulae that are very swollen at the apex, joined by a reduced connective membrane. Female genitalia a pair of fused anal plates and a sternal plate. The body consists of three main parts: the head, thorax and abdomen (Hamidou, H. T. ,2020).

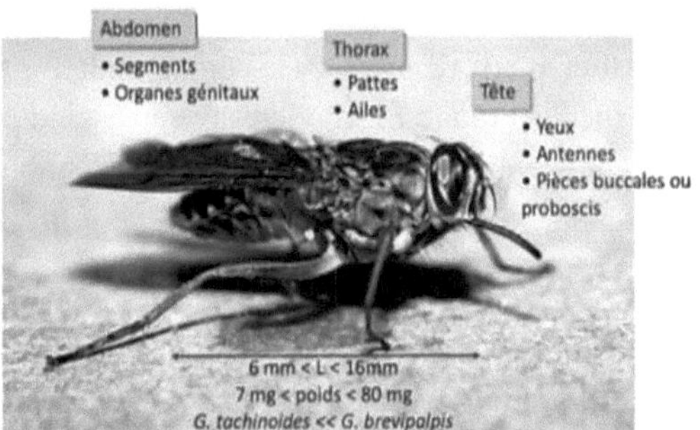

Figure 1: Photo a tsetse fly (source: Pascal Grebault, 2015)

1.3 Biology of tsetse flies

1.3.1 The ecology of tsetse fly

Glossinidae are considered to be highly evolved Diptera, characterised by a unique reproductive cycle. Along with the Hyppoboscidae, Streblidae and Nycteribiidae, they form the puparial group (Itard et Cuisance, 2003) and are the only animal species capable of giving birth to a larva which, without feeding in the external environment, will develop into an adult after pupation. This is made possible by a haematophagous (high-energy) diet. They have an organ similar to the mammalian uterus, which also contains lactiferous glands enabling the larvae to be "suckled" in utero. Most species of tsetse fly during the day, and their movements are limited to searching for food, resting places and females for the males. A tsetse fly for around thirty to fifty minutes a day for males and only five minutes for females (Bouyer, 2009). Tsetse fly therefore spend most of their time in their resting places, which are the undersides of branches or twigs, holes, the undersides of large tree roots and, generally speaking, places that are fairly close to the ground. Several climatic factors (temperature, humidity or hygrometry and light) influence the life of tsetse flies. At temperatures below 16-17°C, tsetse flies cannot lead a normal active life. At temperatures above 38°C, lethal lesions are produced in adults, and pupae cannot withstand temperatures of 32°C. The minimum temperature for pupae to develop normally should not be below 16°C (Pollock, 1982). The hygrometric optimum varies from 50% to 60% for savannah species and from 65% to 85% for forest and forest gallery species (ltard, 1986).

1.3.2 Tsetse fly nutrition

In tsetse flies, both sexes are haematophagous, with preferences varying according to the species. Males gorge themselves approximately every 4 days, while females take 3 meals during gestation: one immediately preceding the intra-uterine moult between the second and third larval stages, the second at a variable time and the last just after larviposition (Itard et Cuisance 2003). Glossina palpalis gambiensis feeds on the following hosts: monitor lizards and crocodiles, which live permanently near water; cattle and warthogs, which are available from time to time to drink; and humans, when they visit tsetse habitats to fish, wash, chop wood or cultivate gardens near watercourses (Pollock, 1996).

1.3.3 Geographical distribution

Tsetse fly distribution is estimated at 10 million km^2 in intertropical Africa (Moloo, 1993). Tsetse flies are found between 15th parallel North and 30th parallel South in East Africa and 20th parallel South in West and Central Africa. The tsetse distribution area is not uniform, and there are vast regions where tsetse are unknown, particularly in East Africa (Moloo, 1993).

1.3.4 The life cycle of tsetse flies.

Tsetse fly have a long and complex life cycle, comprising a long intra-uterine larval phase (3 larval stages remaining in the uterine position and fed by a lactiferous gland for around 10 days), a larval phase in the external environment lasting just a few hours, followed by rapid pupation at a depth of 2 to 8 cm in the soil. The pupation period, which includes the transformation into an IV larva and then metamorphosis into an adult, is highly variable depending on the temperature (20 to 80 days depending on the season and the species). On average, it lasts 30 days in a farm at 25°C. This period is 2 to 4 days shorter in females (Itard 1986, 2000; Cuisance 2001). Hatching takes place by rupture of the puparium in a circular slit (hence the name Cyclorrhaphes given to tsetse flies), by rhythmic swelling of the ptilinum, which also facilitates emergence from the soil. The ptilinum then reinvaginates, and the fly unfolds its wings, inflates its abdomen and raises its proboscis to a horizontal position. The chitin hardens in a few hours, but the teneral tsetse fly ("tener" = tender), which flies away quickly, is still fragile. Its vitality depends on its remaining fat reserves, which in turn depend on the abundance of food hosts for its mother, and the duration of pupation. The first blood meal will be used to develop musculature during an "immature" phase lasting 7 days in the male and 10 days in the female. The female mates before 4 days and generally refuses to mate thereafter, storing the sperm in two spermathecae. This observation led to the use of the sterile male technique, which consists of releasing laboratory-reared and irradiated males in quantities at least equal to or greater than 10 times those of wild males, after the initial reduction of the wild population using conventional techniques (Cuisance and Itard 1973; Cuisance et al., 1979; Cuisance et al., 1984). The first larvisation occurs around day 18th, then every 10 to 11 days, the interval decreasing with temperature (0.5 d/°C). The abortion rate is low in natural conditions (1.6 to 1.9%) and increases with stress (Cuisance, 2001).

Females live longer than males and records 7 to 9 months have been recorded in G. palpalis under natural conditions. However, lifespans are generally less than 80 days and the average number of offspring per female is 5 or 6 days, which is very low. The size of the offspring decreases with the rank of the litter (De Deken et al., 1997), and with the harshness of the environmental conditions, while small tsetse are less resistant to thermal and hygrometric stress (Buxton, 1955).

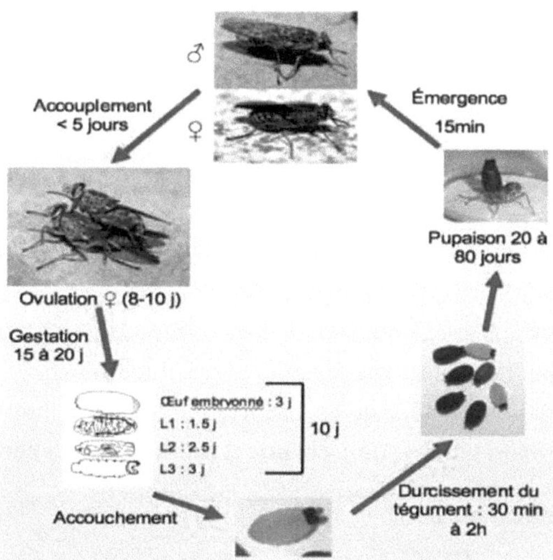

Figure 2: Diagram of the tsetse fly development cycle.
Photo credit: J. Janelle, 2004

1.4 Economic impact of tsetse fly in Africa

In Africa, the direct and indirect impacts of tsetse fly and trypanosomosis cause an estimated annual loss of 4.5 billion dollars. The impacts include reduced livestock productivity, human migration, negative effects on livestock management, but also on agricultural production, land use, the functioning of ecosystems and human well-being. Tsetse flies and trypanosomiasis affect human health, livestock health and rural development across the continent, making a key challenge for rural development in Africa. African trypanosomoses represent a major group of parasitoses that affect both humans and animals. They are caused by trypanosomes, transmitted mainly by tsetse flies (Diptera: Glossinidae). In humans, the disease inevitably leads to death if left untreated. While sleeping sickness is one of today's neglected diseasesAfrican Animal Trypanosomoses (AAT) affecting livestock represent a major obstacle to the development of sustainable agriculture in the humid and sub-humid zones of sub-Saharan Africa. Some 60 million ruminants are at risk (FAO, 2002). The direct consequences of the disease include reduced milk and meat production, mortality, weight gain, draught animal yields and the costs of control programmes, estimated at between US$600 million and US$1.2 billion per year (FAO, 1994). The indirect effects of the disease on livestock are examined in terms of animal traction, breed choice, herd size and structure, and migration.

1.5 Control methods

Tsetse flies are both vectors and reservoirs of trypanosomes (Solano et al., 2018). Vector control makes it possible to reduce trypanosome transmission by reducing the density of flies and, at the same time, eliminating part of the TAA reservoir. This strategy makes perfect sense given the absence of a vaccine and the difficulties associated with other methods of combating TAA. Some authors consider it to be the most sustainable way of eliminating trypanosomoses (Bouyer et al., 2010). IPM can be carried out using a number of methods, divided into two main groups: **non-chemical methods and chemical methods.**

1.5.1 Non-chemical methods

They include ecological control, biological control, mechanical control and genetic control.

Ecological control: this consists of destroying the tsetse fly's habitat by thinning out the forest and felling wild feeding hosts, which are the tsetse fly's preferred hosts. These techniques were successful in their day, but were abandoned in the 1970s, mainly because of the harmful ecological consequences (Solano et al., 2018). It has proved ineffective insofar as tsetse fly, in the absence of their preferred hosts to which they are denied access, are able to adapt to animals of other species in order to feed on their blood, thus increasing the number of animal species that have to be destroyed. This expensive, environmentally destructive and moderately effective method is unacceptable today, as more effective and environmentally friendly means are available.

Biological control: this involves the use of natural predators and parasites of tsetse fly. These are mainly insects: spiders, diptera (azilidae) and fossorial wasps predate adult tsetse flies; ants, birds and mongooses predate pupae. Nematodes and arthropods are parasites of adults (Atrevy, 1978) while certain

Hymenoptera and Diptera parasites of pupae (Bussieras and Chermette, 1991). The effectiveness of this control method requires that the enemy organisms and target insects do not belong to the same geographical or ecological area (Leak, 1999). This method has no practical application at present. Research is focusing on Bacillus sp. and its toxins, which are thought to be used to regulate tsetse fly populations. This bacterium and its toxins have no effect on vertebrates or non-target arthropods (Maillard et Provost, 1975).

Mechanical control: this consists of setting traps or screens impregnated with insecticide, such as the biconical trap (Chalier and Laveissière, 1973), the Vavoua monoconic trap (Laveissière and Grébaut, 1990), the Lancien monoconic trap (Lancien, 1981) and the screen of Laveissière et al, 1987.

Genetic control by sterilisation: this consists of releasing males that have been physically sterilised by gamma radiation or chemically sterilised with aphoxide or metaphoxide. When tsetse fly density is significantly reduced following the use of the methods described above in isolated areas that have not been subject to reinvasion, the sterile insect technique is used to eradicate tsetse "by releasing sterile males". This is the most widely used biological method. It is based the fact that, in principle, female flies will only accept one mating. If this mating is carried out with a sterile male, the female will never produce offspring (Solano et al., 2018). This is a specific and non-polluting technique. Male tsetse flies are sterilised chemically or by ionising radiation (e.g. X-rays) before being released in large numbers. It has been used to eliminate tsetse on the island of Zanzibar and has been in use in Senegal since 2013 (Solano et al., 2018). This method has given very good results in the agropastoral area of Sidéradougou in Burkina Faso (Hargrove and Langley, 1990), but the need for mass production and the use of radioactivity make it difficult to implement and its effectiveness is not immediate (Bouyer et al., 2009, Solano et al., 2018, Vreysen et al., 2013).

1.5.2 Chemical methods

Numerous methods can be used for chemical control:

Ground spraying with residual **insecticides**, which should last longer than the pupation period, was the most widely used method from 1945 until the 1970s. This method is slow and can lead to problems of temporary pollution (Cuisance, 1992). What's more, the cost of such a method is high and the molecules used (dichlorodiphenyltrichloroethane (DDT), dieldrin) have been condemned by fund bailiffs1 because of their persistence and therefore their possible accumulation in trophic chains; as a result, residual treatments, whether by land or by air, have almost completely disappeared.

Sequential spraying with non-slash **aerosols** has been used in flat, open savannah areas. Large areas have been cleaned up (Nigeria, Zimbabwe, Cameroon), but few have been saved because of reinvasions. They consist of five to six night-time treatments spaced ten to fifteen days apart. They are only possible in areas with open vegetation, which are not hilly, and where there is a sufficient temperature inversion at night to allow the insecticide droplets to penetrate the vegetation at the tsetse fly's nocturnal resting places. Despite their great effectiveness, the conditions under which these methods are applied mean that they are rarely used today.

Impregnated traps and screens: from 1974 onwards, the abandonment of residual insecticides and advances in knowledge of tsetse biology, particularly visual and olfactory attractants, gave trapping a leading role, reinforced by the advent of synthetic pyrethroids (lightning contact effect). These methods are now widely used, and a whole range of more or less specific traps and fabric screens (blue/black) are available. The traps can be impregnated with insecticide or sterilising molecules (juvenile hormone mimetics or moult inhibitors). These traps have brought great progress (simple, rapid, non-polluting method) but are subject to major constraints in terms of installation and maintenance.

Several authors have described the good results obtained with these methods of trapping and impregnating screens (Laveissière et al, 1980; Dagnogo and Gouteux, 1983; Mérot et al, 1984; Mawuena and Yacnambe, 1988; Lancien, 1991; Cuisance et al, 1994). However, these measures do not generally lead to the eradication of tsetse, but rather to their control, and it will therefore be necessary to maintain a very long-term approach.

The effectiveness of such methods varies from one tsetse species to another; impregnations have to be renewed and the equipment is vulnerable to theft, wear and tear, and destruction by the weather or animals. In addition, traps are much less attractive to tsetse than cattle. So, if tsetse flies are strongly attracted to livestock, the latter can act as "live traps".

Insecticide impregnation: in the veterinary field, insecticide impregnation of livestock coats transforms livestock into "live traps" (by bathing, spraying, pour-on application or epicutaneous treatment). This method, which is highly effective against most biting arthropods, is very popular with African livestock farmers. For tsetse fly control, Pour On applications are a good complement to other control methods such as insecticide-impregnated screens and/or traps. They are well received by farmers, who can quickly see that they are effective, which facilitates their adoption (Bouyer et al., 2004).

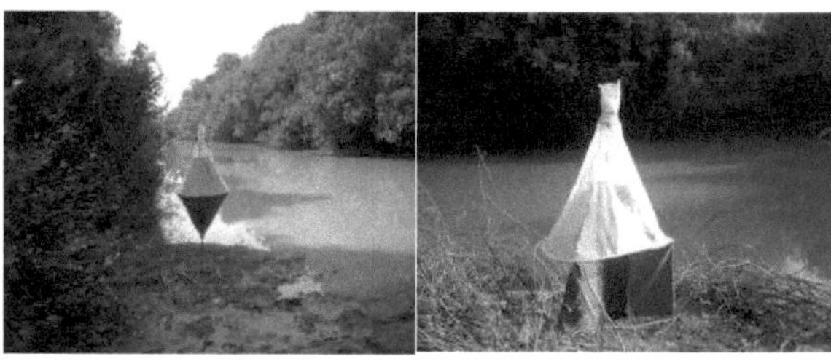

The Challier Laveissière bi-conical trap (1973)

The Vavoua monoconic trap (1990)

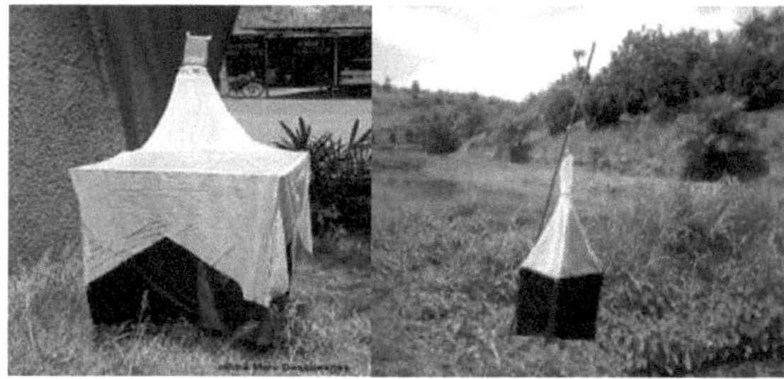

The Dripping Screen trap (1986)
The Lancien monoconic trap (1981)

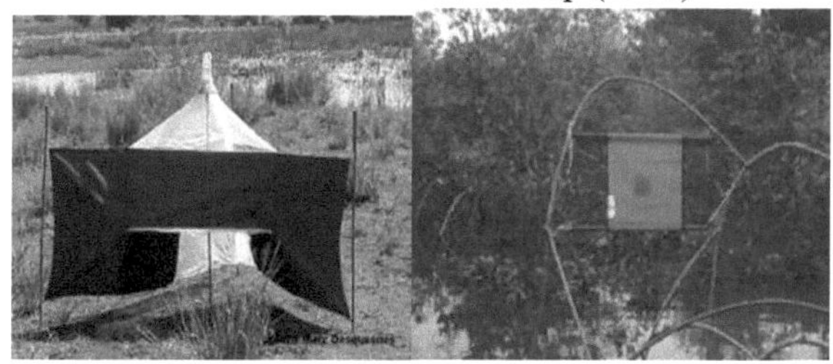

The Nzi trap (1996)

Reduced screen

Figure 3: Control using impregnated traps and screens. Source: (Salou et Rayaisse., 2019)

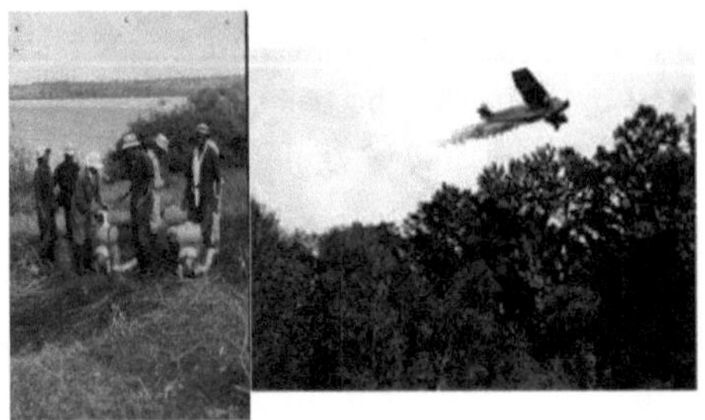

Ground spraying
Aerial spraying

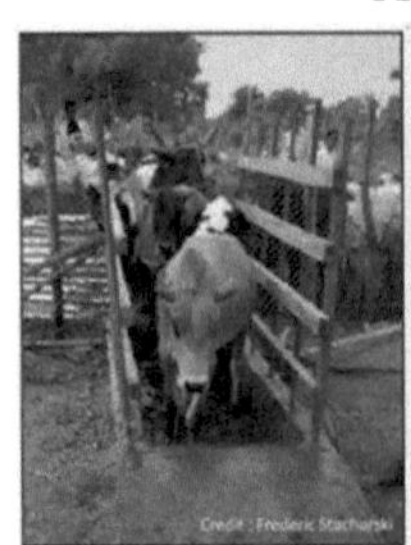

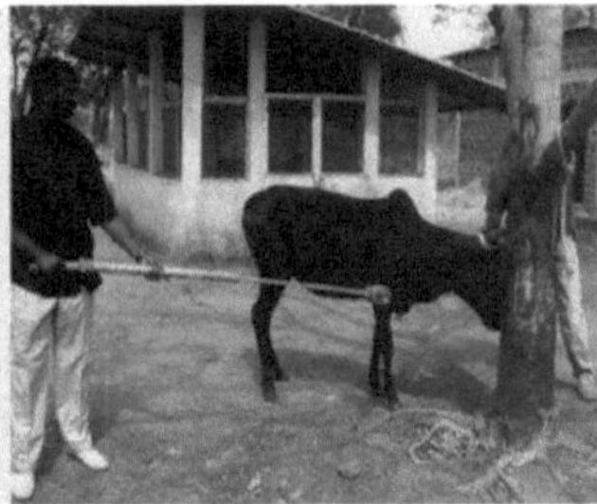

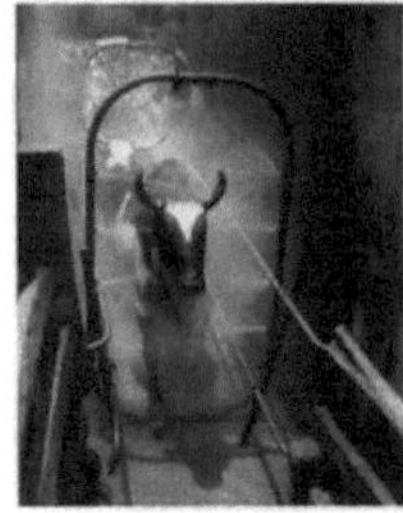

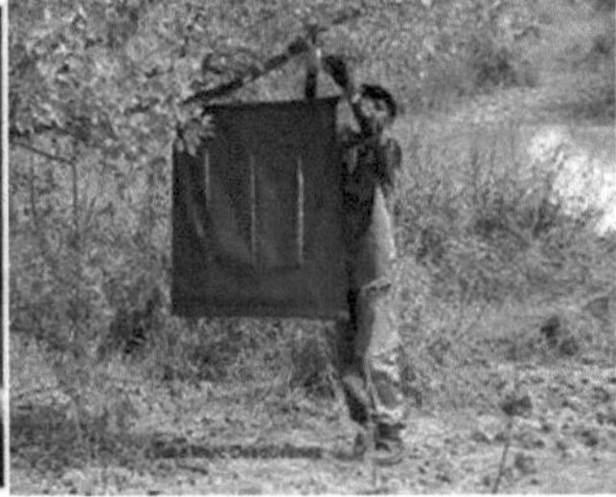

Foot bath Spraying For on Bath insecticide
Screen impregnated insecticide
Figure 4: Direct control. Source: (Salou and Rayaisse, 2019)

2 General information on essential oils

2.1 Definition of essential oils

The term "essential oils" is a generic term for the highly volatile liquid components of plants, marked by a strong, characteristic odour. Essential oils contain a considerable number of biochemical families (hemotypes), including alcohols, phenols, esters, oxides, coumarins, sesquiterpenesterpenols, ketones and aldehydes (https://www.clicours.com/extraction-des-hes-par-hydrodistillation-and-yield/). As you can see, they are not made up of fatty acids or any other fatty substance. It is important to distinguish between essential oils and vegetable oils. Essential oils are by definition secondary metabolites produced by plants as a means of defence against phytophagous pests. Essential oils are obtained by expression (reserved for citrus fruits) or by steam distillation. Terpenes (mainly monoterpenes) make up the majority (around 90%) of these components. These extracts contain an average of 20 to 60 compounds, most of which are not very complex molecules (such as monoterpenes and sesquiterpenes). It is recognised that the effect of these pure compounds may be different from that obtained from plant extracts. They are volatile and soluble in alcohol and oil, but not in water.

Aloysia citrodora

Kingdom: Plantae **Division:**Magnoliophyta **Class:** Magnoliopsida **Order:** Lamiales **Family:** Verbanaceae **Genus:** Aloysia

Figure 5:Aloysia citriodora

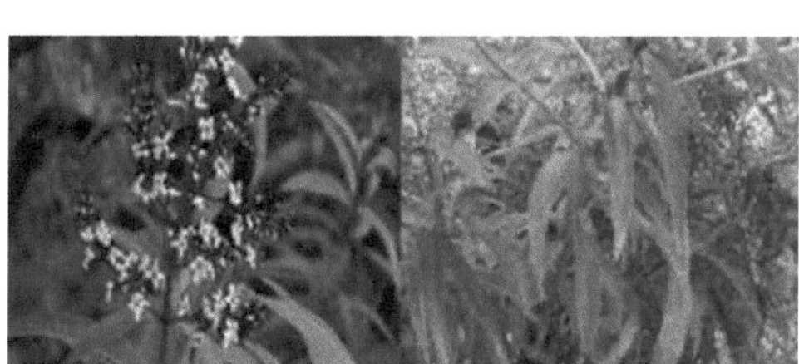

Source : Image.google.fr

Species: Aloysia citriodora Palau, 1784

Fragrant verbena, Aloysia citriodora, is a perennial subshrub of the Verbenaceae family (Lenoir, 2011) measuring 1.50 to 3.00 m in height (De Figueiredo et al., 2002). The stems are angular, fluted with straight, branched branches (Cheurfa et Allem, 2015), bearing pale green, elongated leaves that are 3 to 7 centimetres long and 1 to 2 centimetres wide, whorled in threes or fours on the stems, with very short petioles, rough to the touch. They give off a characteristic lemon scent when crumpled. The long flowers, arranged in spikes, have four petals fused at the base into a tube and spread out in four bicoloured lobes: white on the outside and purplish blue on the inside (Ghédira and Goetz, 2017).

Lantana Camara L. (Lantana) Kingdom: Plantae

Division: Magnoliophyta
Class: Magnoliopsida

Order: Lamiales **Family:** Verbanaceae **Genus:** Lantana
Species : Lantana camara

Figure 6:Lantana camara

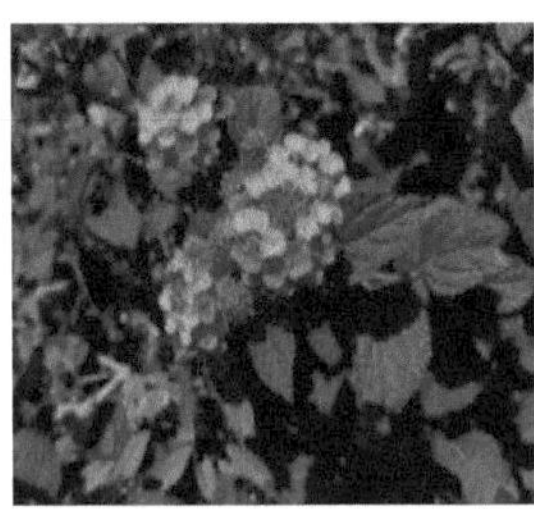

Source : Image.google.fr

Lantana is a small, bushy evergreen shrub in the Verbenaceae family, native to tropical regions, particularly western India. It is adapted to subtropical or tropical climates, but can also be grown in milder climates (Huynh, 2009), and comprises around 150 species (Ghisalberti, 2000).

Eucalyptus camaldulensis

Kingdom : Plantae
Division: Magnoliophyta **Class:** Magnoliopsida **Order:** Myrtales
Family: Myrtacae
Genus: Eucalyptus
Species: Eucalyptus camaldulensis Dehnh, 1832

Figure 7:Eucalyptus camaldulensis

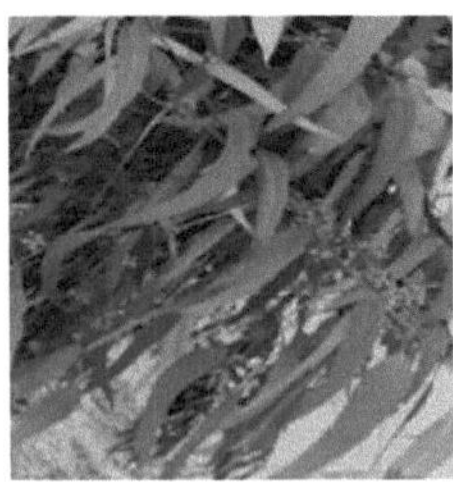

Source : Image.google.fr

The Eucalyptus is a very beautiful tree, 30 to 35 m tall and up to 100 m in its natural environment (Traore, 1991). Eucalyptus trees have evergreen, leathery, hairless leaves, which vary according to the age of the branches. Young twigs have broad, short leaves, Opposite, sessile, oval, blue-white and waxy, with a true ribbed blade. Older twigs: have aromatic, falcate leaves, 12 to 30 cm long, narrow, pointed, thick, dark green, short-stalked, alternate and hanging vertically (Goetz and Ghedira, 2012).

Hyptis suaveolens

Kingdom : Plantae
Division: Magnoliophyta **Class:** Magnoliopsida **Order:** Lamiales **Family:** Lamiacea
Genus : Hyptis

Species: Hyptis suaveolens (L.) Poit, 1806

Figure 8: Hyptis suaveolens

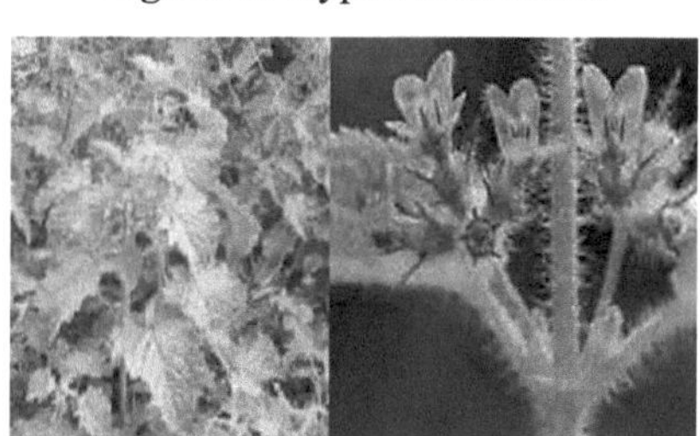

Source : Image.google.fr

Hyptis suaveolens is a highly aromatic herb that grows to around 2 m in height (Parsons Cuthbertson, 1992). It generally grows in open areas and well-drained soils. In the Sudanian region, it is sometimes found on roadsides, around villages and on crops during the first years of fallow (Kerharo, 1974).

Cymbopogon citratus

The systematic position of Cymbopogon citratus is as follows:

Kingdom : Plantae
Division: Magnoliophyta **Class:** Liliopsida **Order:** Cyperales **Family:** Poacae
Genre: Cymbogon
Species: Cymbopogon citratus (DC.) Staf, 1906

Figure 9:Cymbopogon citratus

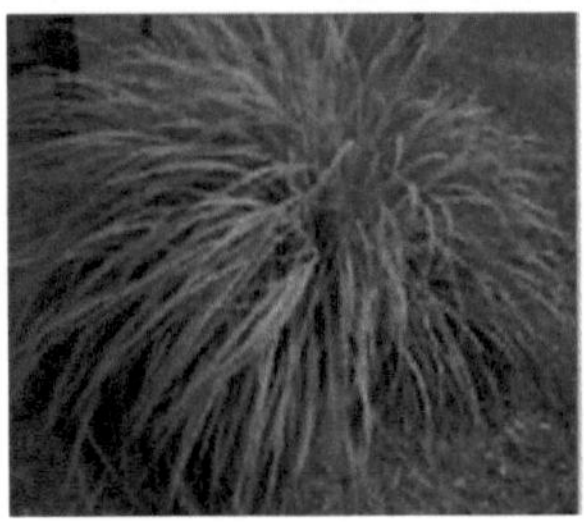

Source : Image.google.fr

Lemongrass C. citratus belongs to the Poaceae family, which comprises around 660 genera and 9,000 species (Clayton, 1968). C. citratus is a perennial, unbranched, lemon-scented herb growing in dense clumps. Leaves are isolated, light green, pubescent, strongly scented, long-tapered, sheath-like for part of their length, with hyaline margins formed by numerous small teeth directed towards the apex; the underground part consists of a bulb or rhizome. Flowering stem with numerous branches ending in greenish clusters of spikes. Reproduction is by rhizomes (Nacoulma OG, 1996).

Mentha piperita

The systematic position of Mentha piperita Linné, 1753 is as follows:

Kingdom: Plantae **Division:** Angiosperm **Class:** Magnoliopsida **Order:** Lamiales **Family:** Lamiaceae
Genus : Mentha
Species: Mentha piperita (Linné, 1753).

Figure 10:Mentha piperita

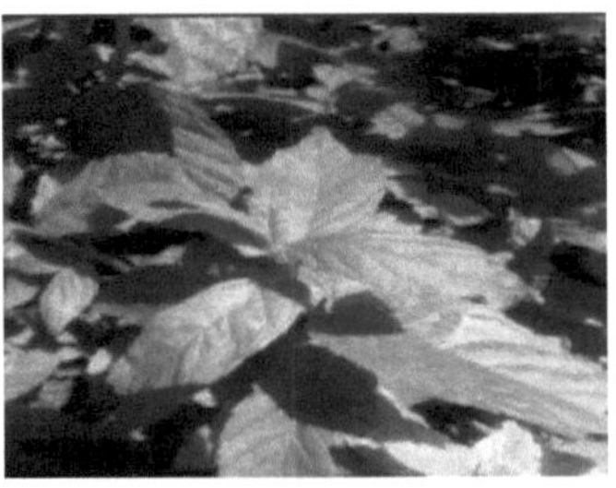

Source : Image.google.fr

Mints, from the Latin name Mentha, are perennial, herbaceous, indigenous and very fragrant plants belonging to the Lamiaceae family (Jahandiez et Maire, 1932). Since ancient times, mints have been used in an infinite variety of and play a major role in therapeutics. As a diffusible stimulant and also a diffusible sedative, Mint is highly effective against nervousness and various nervous symptoms. In terms of chemical principles, most Mint species owe their odour and activity to their essential oils or Mint Essences (Il Idrissi, 1982). Peppermint is a perennial plant with a rhizome that clings to the ground and spreads by stolons. Its leaves are 4 to 10 cm long, oval, dark green, with reddish tints in the sun and coppery red in the shade. They are covered with large, rounded secretory hairs in which volatile odorous substances accumulate. The stems are purplish and square in cross-section (Bruneton, 2009).

2.2 Insecticidal activity of essential oils: mechanisms of action .

Relatively little is known about the mode action of essential oils in insects (Bekele et al., 2001; Isman, 2000). Essential oils have a physiological effect on insects through their antiappetent effects, affecting the growth, moulting, fecundity and development of insects and mites. Work by Keane et al (1999) has shown that mono terpenes inhibit cholinesterase. Essential oils are thought to act physically directly on the cuticle of soft-bodied arthropods. Isman (2000) makes this hypothesis because several essential oils appear to be more effective on soft-bodied arthropods. Octopamine is a neuromodulator specific to invertebrates: this molecule has a regulatory effect on the heartbeat, motricity, ventilation, flight and metabolism of invertebrates. Enan (2000) and Isman (2000) linked application of eugenol, alpha- terpineol and cinnamic alcohol to the blocking of octopamine acceptor sites. Enan (2005) also demonstrated an effect tyramine, another insect neurotransmitter. In general, essential oils are known to be acute neurotoxicants that interfere with octopaminergic transmitters in arthropods. These oils are therefore not very toxic to warm-blooded animals.

2.3 History the use of essential oils

Known for their powerful therapeutic properties and used for thousands of years in China, India, the Middle East, Egypt, Greece, Latin America (Aztecs, Mayas, Incas) and Africa, essential oils were forgotten in the Middle Ages (https://cyrusmagnetiseur.jimdofree.com/aromath%C3%A9rapie/). At this point, Europe experienced a return to barbarism, with a general decline in knowledge. It was not until the arrival of the Arabs that plant-based medicine began to flourish once again, with plants once again taking pride of place in the therapeutic arsenal of the time. Plant extracts have long been used as insecticides. In certain regions of black Africatobacco leaves mixed with water were used combat mosquitoes. In Morocco, the use of plants against mosquito invasions is a very common practice, especially in rural areas.

PART TWO
OUR STUDY

3 Research question and hypothesis

3.1 Questions for research

What are the effects of essential oils on tsetse fly?
Which textile support ensures the best persistence of the active ingredients in essential oils?

3.2 Hypotheses of research

Essential oils have insecticidal properties against tsetse flies.
Whatman papers ensure that the active ingredients in essential oils last longer.

3.3 Aims of the study

3.3.1 General objective

The general aim of this study is to assess the efficacy of essential oils in protecting livestock against tsetse flies, the vectors of animal trypanosomes.

3.3.2 Specific objectives

The specific objectives of the study are :

- Laboratory testing of the toxicity of essential oils on Glossina palpalis gambiensis adults;
- Find a textile support that ensures better persistence of the active ingredients of essential oils in the laboratory.

4 Materials and methods

4.1 Material used

The biological material used consisted of tsetse flies and essential oils. The tsetse flies used were Glossina palpalis gambiensis, Vanderplanck (1949) from the CIRDES insectarium. The tsetse flies were 1 day old males, all teneral (having not yet taken a blood meal after leaving the puparium). The choice of males was motivated by the requirements of the insectarium, females being necessary for the maintenance of the colony. This subspecies was chosen for this study because of its epidemiological importance in West Africa. They are mainly vectors of animal trypanosomes (Trypanosoma vivax, Trypanosoma congolense, Trypanosoma brucei brucei) but also of the human trypanosome (Trypanosoma brucei gambiense) (Pollock, 1996).Essential oils were tested in the present study because of their increasingly proven efficacy as insecticides and insect repellents. The essential oils were obtained by hydrodistillation using a Clevenger-type apparatus from the dry leaves, separately, and then from their mixture in mass proportions of 80% and 20%. These essential oils were supplied by the laboratory of chemistry and natural substances at Nazi Boni University. A total of 09 essential oils of equal concentration were tested.

Figure 11: Glossins / essential oils in the refrigerator.

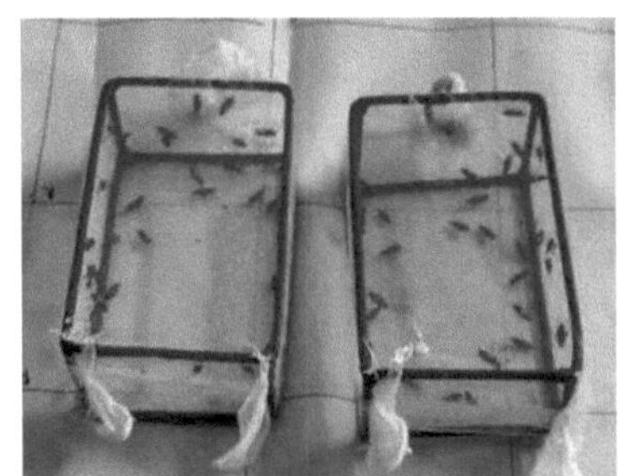

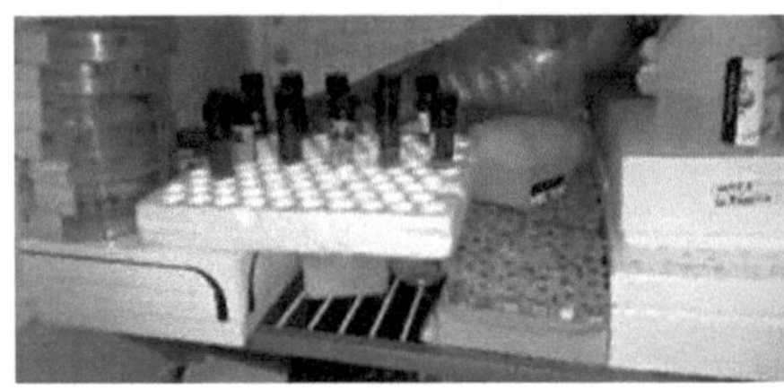

Source: Clichée Julien October 2022

The technical equipment consisted of Roubaud cages, soft forceps, coverslips (Menzel.Glazer ; Deckglaser/cover slips ; 18x18m), glass microfibre paper (labware, ref.FMVA47, Dim 47mm) , grease-free filter paper (elvetec service ; ref.0032A00009, Dim: 150mm) , Gilson type micropipette (pipetman 1 to 20ul), alcohol 90°C, pairs of gloves, a thermo-hygrometer, an air conditioner, a refrigerator, a stopwatch and CO2 gas.

4.2 Methodology

4.2.1 Evaluation of the efficacy of essential oils on teneral males of Glossina palpalis gambiensis in the laboratory. Before each manipulation, the flies were transported from the insectarium to the test room, where they were anaesthetised with CO2 for 30 seconds and immediately exposed to distilled water (negative control), essential oils (treatments) and a piece of screen impregnated with insecticide (positive control). The tarsal contact time was 5 seconds; this corresponds to the average contact time between tsetse flies and traps and screens observed in the field (Laveissière et al., 1985). The rate of Knock Down (KD) tsetse flies, i.e. those knocked out, was assessed at different times (30 min, 1 h, 2 h, 3 h, 4 h, 6 h) and the mortality rate at 24 h after exposure. For each test solution, 20 male flies were used and the test was repeated 3 times. The tests were carried out under laboratory conditions. The temperature was checked daily and remained fairly constant at around 27+/-2°C. Humidity was 85%.

❖ Topical application of essential oils to the back of the chest:

A 1µl microdrop of crude oil was applied to the dorsal surface of the thorax of each fly. Tsetse flies were treated individually by micropipette.

❖ Forced contact of Glossina palpalis gambiensis on the lamellae:

We deposited 5µl of crude oil onto 3.24cm^2 of the coverslip, then using the soft forceps, each anaesthetised fly was brought into contact with the tarsally-treated coverslip for 5 seconds.

❖ Forced contact of Glossina palpalis gambiensis on glass microfibre paper and ash-free filter paper:

We impregnated the microfibre paper with 20ul of crude oil over 7.38 cm^2 and the ash-free degreasing filter paper with 20ul of crude oil over 3.57cm^2, then using soft forceps, each anaesthetised fly was brought into contact with the paper treated by the tarsi for 5 seconds.

4.2.2 Study sites

Our work was carried out in the parasitology laboratory of the Centre International de Recherche-Développement sur l'Elevage en Zone Subhumide (CIRDES). CIRDES is an intergovernmental organisation created by replacing the Centre de Recherches sur les Trypanosomoses Animales, following the signing of a convention in December 1991, which was ratified by the Ministers in charge of Livestock of the five member countries of the Conseil de l'Entente (Benin, Burkina Faso, Côte d'Ivoire, Niger and Togo). Other countries joined later, including Mali in 2002, Guinea Bissau in 2005 and Guinea in 2013. It has financial and administrative autonomy and international legal personality, and signed a headquarters agreement with Burkina Faso on 12 August 1997. Ghana and France are associated countries of CIRDES. Its areas of activity are: improving animal health and production; conserving animal genetic resources; preserving the environment; sustainable integrated management of agro-sylvo-pastoral resources; training, exchanges and technology transfer.

Type and period of study

This prospective study ran from [1]August 2022 to 31 January 2023.

Study population

Our study population consisted of Glossina palpalis gambiensis that met the following criteria:

Inclusion

All tsetse flies were included in the study: males, day-olds and general.

Non-inclusion criteria

Not all tsetse flies were included in this study:

Male, one day old, general who can't fly.

Sample size and Sampling

A total of 20 1-day-old adult tsetse flies were used for each solution tested. The sampling technique consisted of selecting tsetse flies that met the eligibility criteria during the study period.

Statistical analysis

All the data were first recorded, organised and summarised in Microsoft Excel 2010. Statistical analyses were performed using the non-parametric Kaplan-Meier estimator, the Cox model (Cox, 1972), the Pearson Chi-square test and the Wilcoxson test R software (version 4.2.2.) at the 5% threshold. Where the treatment was significant, multiple pairwise comparisons were carried out using the (glht) function in the (multcomp) package.

5 Results

5.1 Effectiveness of essential oils applied topically to the back of the chest:

In the case of the application of essential oils to the dorsal surface of the thorax of Glossina palpalis gambiensis, whatever the essential oil, the knock-down rate was 100%. 24 hours later, we recorded a mortality rate of 100% whatever the essential oil. No effect was observed in the control batch during exposure.

5.2 Efficacy of essential oils after forced contact with Glossina palpalis gambiensis on treated strips.

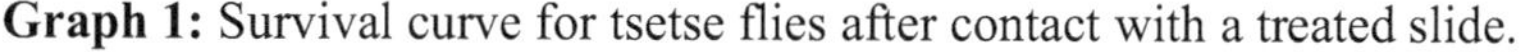

Graph 1: Survival curve for tsetse flies after contact with a treated slide.

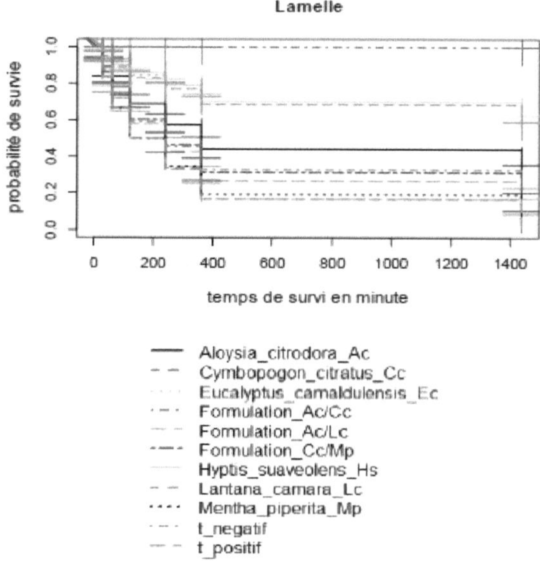

The results showed that there was a significant difference (P =<2e-16 < 0.05) between all essential oils tested and the controls. A general analysis of the results showed that 30 minutes, 1h, 2h, 4h, 6h, after forced contact of Glossina palpalis gambiensis on the slide, we recorded a knock down rate of between 20% and 100%. Twenty-four hours after Glossina palpalis gambiensis was forced onto the slide, we recorded a mortality rate of between 20% and 95% for all the essential oils.

5.3 Effectiveness of essential oils after forced contact with Glossina palpalis gambiensis on microfibre paper.

Graph 2: Tsetse fly survival curve after contact with treated fibre paper.

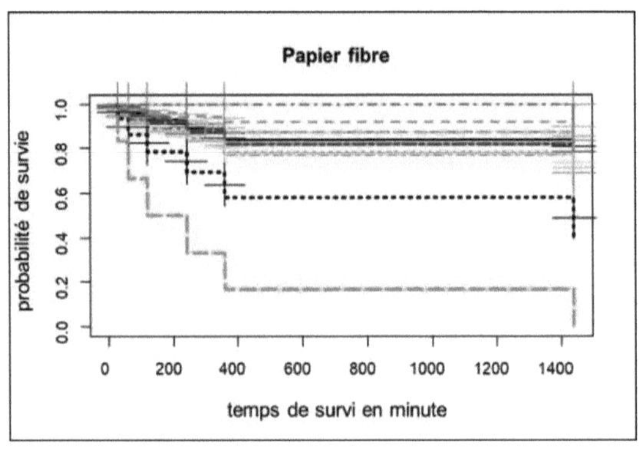

Aloysia_citrodora_Ac
Cymbopogon_citratus_Cc
Eucalyptus_camaldulensis_Ec
Formulation_Ac/Cc
Formulation_Ac/Lc
Formulation_Cc/Mp
Hyptis_suaveolens_Hs
Lantana_camara_Lc
Mentha_piperita_Mp
t_negatif
t_positif

The results showed that there was a significant difference (p=< 2.2e-16 < 0.05) between all the essential oils tested and the controls. A general analysis of the results shows that 30 minutes, 1h, 2h, 4h, 6h, after forced contact of Glossina palpalis gambiensis on glass microfibre paper, we recorded a knock down rate of between 5% and 40%. Twenty-four hours after forced contact with Glossina palpalis gambiensis on the glass microfibre paper, we recorded a mortality rate of between 5% and 50% for all the essential oils.

5.4 Efficacy of essential oils after forced contact with Glossina palpalis gambiensis on filter paper without degreasing agents

No effect (KD effect and lethal effect) was observed in tsetse flies after contact with filter paper without degreasing agents, whatever the essential oil.

6 Discussion

6.1 Evaluation of the efficacy of essential oils on teneral males of Glossina palpalis gambiensis in the laboratory.

In our study, the essential oils of all the plants were found to be highly toxic by topical application and forced contact on the lamellae against the teneral males of Glossina palpalis gambiensis. In fact, several previous studies have demonstrated the effectiveness of the oil from these plants against insects and fungi. The results of the study by Khani et al (2012) suggest that the essential oil of Aloysia citriodora could be used as a potential control agent against C. maculatus and T. confusum. Results obtained by (Tia et al., 2019) show that C. citratus essential oil is toxic to C. puncticollis. The finding by Rajashekar et al (2012) indicated that methanol extract of Lantana camara leaves was toxic to S. oryzae, C. chinensis and T. castaneum, showing that Lantana camara leaves are becoming a potential source of biopesticide for stored grain pest control strategies. Work by Koroghli, K. (2018) showed that the M. piperita essential oil tested exerts significant inhalation toxicity on Rhyzopertha dominica adults. Work carried out on the essential oil of H. suaveolens revealed that the essential oil of this plant effectively repels mosquitoes and can be used as a vector control agent against malaria (Abagli et al., 2010; Jaenson et al., 2006). Somda et al (2007) demonstrated the antifungal properties of Taiwanese E. camaldulensis essential oils against ten fungal species. Several studies have shown that the toxicity of essential oils is influenced by their chemical composition. This generally depends on the origin, climatic conditions, method and period of extraction and the part of the plant (Manal et al., 2013). The toxic effects of these essential oils could depend on their chemical compositions and the insect's level of sensitivity (Casida J.H., 1990). On the other hand, the essential oils in our study showed weak insecticidal activity by forced contact on glass microfibre paper and no insecticidal activity by forced contact on grease-free filter paper at the doses tested against teneral males of Glossina palpalis gambiensis; this leads us to think that the active principle contained in the essential oils would probably be absorbed by the paper. The high mortality and knock down rate can be explained by the speed of penetration and the amount of essential oil absorbed through the insect cuticle. Our results are in agreement with those of Bass et al, 2016 (100%) using a concentration of 4- 8% of neem oil on Glossina palpalis gambiensis by topical applications on the dorsal surface of the thorax. In contrast to the high mortality rates we obtained, low mortality rates were recorded elsewhere using a formulation of azadirachtin on Glossina fuscipes fuscipes (Makoundou et al, 1995). The difference between our results is due on the one hand to the species and on the other hand because a commercial formulation of azadirachtin was used on Glossina fuscipes fuscipes, instead of pure oil. The high mortality and knock-down observed with topical applications of the essential oils to the dorsal surface of the thorax leads us to believe that the essential oils tested could be used to control tsetse flies in the residual treatment of tsetse resting places (tree trunks and branches), taking into account the dose. The insecticidal activity of the plant combinations would be due to the combined toxic effect of the major compounds of the oils taken individually. Recently, Wangrawa et al (2022) have shown that the improvement of essential oils by combinations is due to the appearance of new compounds previously absent in the individual oils.

6.2 Limits of the study

The main limitation of our study related to the study population. Our research focused only on the insecticide effect and exclusively on teneral males of Glossina palpalis gambiensis. In the future, it would be interesting to supplement this work with :

- Study of impact of essential oils on the reproductive potential of these species of tsetse fly.

- Study of repellent effect of these essential oils on adult males and females tsetse species tested.

CONCLUSION

Studies of the insecticidal properties of essential oils have shown them to be effective against Glossina palpalis gambiensis. The results obtained from topical applications give reason to hope that all the essential oils can be used in the field as a direct spray on tsetse flies. The high mortality and knock-down rates observed by forced tarsal contact on the lamella suggest that certain essential oils could be used for residual treatment of tsetse fly resting places (tree trunks and branches) and for impregnation of lures (traps and screens). The results obtained by forced tarsal contact on glass microfibre paper and a grease-free filter do not allow us to envisage the use of all the essential oils in the field, given the dose that would have to be applied to achieve a high mortality rate. However, in the context of a field application with view to exploiting the insecticidal effect, other studies would be useful. These include persistence on the coat, appropriate formulation, cost of use, toxicity to livestock, and residues in milk and meat. Although this laboratory study showed an interesting insecticidal effect for all the essential oils, a field trial seems necessary to study this same efficacy under natural conditions.

REFERENCES

Abagli and Alavo J. Appl. Biosci. 2020. Insect repellent potentialities of coarse balsam, Hyptis suaveolens Poit. (Lamiaceae): Prospects for mosquito control in tropical areas.

Abagli AZ, Alavo TBC, Djouaka R, Ahomadégbé MA, Ahoton LE, Yayi E, Avlessi F. 2010. Repellency rate of different concentrations of Hyptis suaveolens essential oil against the mosquito Anopheles gambiae (Diptera: Culicidae). Actes du 2ème colloque des Sciences, Cultures et Technologies de l'Université d'Abomey-Calavi (UAC)- Bénin (In press).

Akono, P. N., Belong, P., Tchoumbougnang, F., Bakwo Fils, E.-M., & Fankem, H. (2012). Chemical composition and insecticidal effects of essential oils of fresh leaves of Ocimum canum Sims and Ocimum basilicum L. on adults of Anopheles funestus ss, vector of malaria in Cameroon. Journal of Applied Biosciences, 59, 4340-4348.Spottedà http://www.m.elewa.org/JABS/2012/59/7.pdf%5Cnhttp://m.elewa.org/JABS/2012/59/7.pdf

Atrevy F., 1978. Tsetse flies in the People's Republic of Benin: importance for livestock farming, principles and methods of eradication. Doctorat Vétérinaire thesis, 1978. Inter-State School of Veterinary Science and Medicine, Dakar. 115 pages.

Bauer, B., Amsler-Delafosse, S., Clausen, P.H., Kabore, I., Petrich-Bauer, J., 1995. Successful application of deltamethrin pour on to cattle in a campaign against tsetse flies (Glossina spp.) in the pastoral zone of Samorogouan, Burkina Faso. Trop. Med. Parasitol. 46, 183-189.

Bass, A., Traore, A., Traore, A., Traore, A., Bengaly, S., Diakite, B., & Diarra, C. (2016). Evaluation of the efficacy of the 8% neem oil solution in the control of tsetse flies and African animal trypanosomosis in Mali.

Bastien, F. (2008). Larvicidal effect of essential oils on Stomoxys calcitrans Réunion (Doctoral dissertation).

Bokobana, E. M., Koba, K., Poutouli, W. P., Akantetou, P. K., Nadio, N. A., Laba, B., ... Sanda, K. (2014). Evaluation of the insecticidal and repellent potential of Cymbopogon schoenanthus (L.) spreng essential oil on Aphis gossypii Glover (Homoptera: Aphididae), cotton pest in Togo. Reveue Cames, 2(2), 48-55.

Bekele J. and Hassanali A. ,2001 : Blend effects in the toxicity of the essential oil constituents of Ocimum kilimandscharicum and Ocimum kenyense (Labiatae) on two post-harvest insect pests. Phytochemestry, 57 : 385 - 391.

Bouyer J., Kaboré I., Stachurski F. and Desquesne M., 2004. Control of bovine ectoparasites. Epi cutaneous treatment of cattle. Bobo-Dioulasso: Centre international de recherche- développement sur l'élevage en zone subhumide (CIRDES). Data sheet: 12 pages

Bouyer, F., Bouyer, J., Seck, M., Sall, B., Dicko, A., Lancelot, R., Chia, E. et al. (2015). Importance of vector-borne infections in different production systems: bovine trypanosomosis and the innovation dynamics of livestock producers in senegal', Rev Sci Tech Off Int Epiz **34**, 213-225. 48

Bouyer, J., Balenghien, T., Ravel, S., Vial, L., Sidibé, I., Thévenon, S., Solano, P. and Meeûs, T. D. (2009). Population sizes and dispersal pattern of tsetse flies : rolling on the river Molecular Ecology **18**(13), 2787-2797. _eprint : https ://onlinelibrary.wiley.com/doi/pdf/10.1111/j.1365-294X.2009.04233.x.

Bouyer, J., Ravel, S., Guerrini, L., Dujardin, J.-P., Sidibé, I., Vreysen, M. J. B., Solano, P. and De Meeûs, T. (2010). Population structure of Glossina palpalis gambiensis (Diptera: Glossinidae) between river basins in Burkina Faso: Consequences for area-wide integrated pest management', Infection, Genetics and Evolution 10(2), 321-328.

Bouyer, F. E. (2015). Trypanosomiasis risk and innovation: the case of livestock farmers in West Africa. l'Ouest (Doctoral dissertation, Université Montpellier). URL: https ://www.sciencedirect.com/science/article/pii/S1567134810000043 30, 49

Bouyer, J., Balenghien, T., Ravel, S., Vial, L., Sidibé, I., Thévenon, S., Solano,P. and Meeûs, T. D. (2009). Population sizes and dispersal pattern of tsetse flies : rolling on the river Molecular Ecology 18(13), 2787-2797. _eprint: https : //onlinelibrary.wiley.com/doi/pdf/10.1111/j.1365-294X.2009.04233.x.

Bouyer, J. (2009). Tsetse fly dispersal. Insectes, 153, 21-24.

Bruneton, J. (2009). Mint in: Pharmacognosie, phytochimie, plantes médicinales, 4th edn, Tec & Doc, Paris, pp. 631-638.

Bussieras J. and Chermette R, (1991). Veterinary Parasitology. Entomology. Service de Parasitologie. Ecole Nationale Vétérinaire d'Alfort: Maisons Alfort. 163 pages.

Buxton, P. A. (1955). The natural history of tsetse flies. An account of the biology of the genus Glossina (Diptera). Memory of London School of Hygiene & Tropical Medicine. No. 10, H.K. Lewis, London.

Casida J.H., 1990. Pesticide mode of action, evidence for implications of a finite number of biochemical targets. In: Casida J.E. (ed.). Pesticides and alternatives. Innovative chemical and Biological Approaches to Pest Control. Amsterdam: Elsevier, pp. 11-22.

Carlos, Espinel-Correal (2010). Analysis of evolution of granulovirus populations PhopGV in contact with alternative hosts Phthorimaea operculella and Tecia solanivora (Lepidoptera: Gelechiidae). École Nationale Supérieure des Mines de Saint-Étienne.192p.

Chalier A. and Laveissiere C. (1973). Un nouveau piège pour la capture des glossines (Glossina: Diptera, Muscidae): description et essais sur le terrain. Cahiers ORSTOM. Série Entomologie Médicale et Parasitologie, Il: 251-262.

Cheurfa M and Allem R, 2015. Evaluation of the antioxidant activity of different extracts of Aloysia triphylla leaves. Phytotherapy, 14(3): 181-187.

Clayton, W., 1968. Gramineae. In: Flora of West Africa: Tropical Africa, vol. 3, pp. 349- 512.

Cox D. R, 1972. Regression models and life table. Journal of the Royal Statistical Society, Series B 34: 187-202.

Cuisance, D. and J. Itard. 1973. Release of Glossina tachinoides West sterile males. In a natural site of low density (Bas-Logone, Cameroon). Revue d'Elevage et de Médecine vétérinaire des Pays tropicaux 26(4): 405-422.

Cuisance D., Politzar H., Merot P., Tamboura I., 1984. Release of irradiated males in the integrated tsetse fly control campaign in the pastoral zone of Sideradougou (Burkina Faso). Rev. Elev. Med. Vet. Pays Trop **37**: 449-67.

Cuisance D., Barre N., DE Deken R, (1994). Ectoparasites of animals: ecological, biological, genetic and mechanical control methods. Rev. Scie. Techn. Off. Int. Epiz. 994, 13 (4), 305-] 356.

Cuisance D., (1992). Impact on the environment of tsetse control. Atelier sur les méthodes de recherche en écologie des traitements anti-acridiens en Afrique, C.R. de l'atelier CEE-CIRAD, Montpellier (France), Nov]. 992,] 09]] 6.

Cuisance, D. (2001). Course on tsetse fly and trypanosomiasis for the Advanced Veterinary Studies Certificate in Tropical Pathology. CIRAD-EMVT, Montpellier, France : 102 p

Dagnogo M. and Gouteux J.P., 1983. Field trial of different insecticides against Glossina palpalis (Robineau-Desvoidy) and Glossina tachinoides Westwood.l. Repellent effect of WHO] 998, WHO 2002, WHO 200, WHO 18 and WHO 570. Cahier ORSTOM, ser. Ent. méd.Parasit, 1983, 21 (l), 29-34.
De Figueiredo RO, Stefanini MB, Ming LC, Marques M and Facanali R, 2002. Essential Oil Composition of Aloysia triphylla (L'Herit) Britton Leaves Cultivated in Botucatu, São Paulo, Brazil, page 131-134.

Deken, R. D., Bossche, P. V. D., Sangare, M., Gnanvi, C., Missanda, J. H., & Hees, J. V. (1997). Effect of the life-span of female Glossina palpalis gambiensis on the weight and size of its progeny. Medical and Veterinary Entomology, 11(1), 95-101.

Enan E. 2000: Insecticidal activity of essential oils: octopaminergic sites of action. Comparative Biochemistry and Physiology Part C :Toxicology&Pharmacology. Vol130 (3) Nov 2001, p 325-337.
Felicia Johnson, Kouamé Raphaël, Oussou Coffi, Kanko Zanahi, Félix Tonzibo, Kouahou Foua-Bi, Yao Tano 2018. Bioefficacy of essential oils of three plant species (Ocimum gratissimum, Ocimum canum and Hyptis suaveolens), of the Labiatae family in the control of Sitophilus zeamais. European Journal of Scientific Research ISSN 1450-216X / 1450-202X Vol. 150 No 3, pp. 273-284.

Gimonneau, G., Alioum, Y., Abdoulmoumini, M., Zoli, A., Cene, B., Adakal, H., Bouyer, J., 2016. Insecticide and Repellent Mixture Pour-On Protects Cattle against Animal Trypanosomosis. PLoS Negl. Trop. Dis. 10, 1-16.

Ghédira K and Goetz P, 2017. Sweet verbena Aloysia citriodora Paláu (Lippia citriodora). Phytotherapy, 15(1): 33-37.

Ghisalberti E.L. 2000. Lantana camara L. (Verbenaceae). Fitoterapia, (71):P.467-486.
Gitari, M. W., Akinyemi, S. A., Thobakgale, R., Ngoejana, P. C., Ramugondo, L., Matidza, M., & Nemapate, N. (2018). Physicochemical and mineralogical characterization of Musina mine copper and New Union gold mine tailings: Implications for fabrication of beneficial geopolymeric construction materials. Journal of African Earth Sciences, 137, 218-228.

Goetz, P; Ghedira, K; 2012. Phytotherapie antinfectieuse. [online].Springer .Paris, 147- 180.Available at:https://link.springer.com/chapter/10.1007/978-2-8178-0058- 5_7.

Hamidou, H. T. (2020). Study of host-vector-parasite and symbiont interactions in the control of the Tsetse fly, vector of African Animal Trypanosomiasis in West Africa.

Hargrove J.W. and Langley P.A., 1990. Sterilizing tsetse in the field: a successful triai. Bulletin of Entomological Research/ Volume 80 /Issue 04/ December 1990, pp 397-403.

Hoare, C. A. (1972). The trypanosomes of mammals. A zoological monograph. The trypanosomes of mammals. A zoological monograph.

Huynh T.M.D. 2009. Impacts of heavy metals plant/earthworm interaction.

telluric microflora. PhD in Microbial Ecology. University of Paris-Est. France. P.151.

Il Idrissi, A., (1982). Etude des huiles essentielles de quelques Espèces Salivia, Lavandula et Mentha du Maroc, Thèse de troisième cycle, Université Mohammed V, Faculté des Sciences de Rabat.

Isman, 2000: Plant essential oils for pest and disease management. Crop Protection 19 (2000) 603-60

Itard J., 1986. Tsetse flies. CIRAD -Etudes et synthèses de l'EMVT. Maisons-Alfort: Institut d'élevage et de médecine vétérinaire des pays tropicaux. 155 pages.

Itard, J. (2000). African animal trypanosomoses. In Chartier, C., Itard, J., Morel, P. C., Troncy, P. M. (eds): Précis de Parasitologie vétérinaire tropicale. Universités francophones, AUPELF-UREF, EM inter, Editions TEC & Doc, London-Paris-New York, pp 773.

Itard J. & Cuisance D. (2003). Cyclic vectors of trypanosomoses. In: Principales maladies infectieuses et parasitaires du bétail. Europe et régions chaudes. Generalities, viral diseases. Lefèvre Pierre-Charles, Blancou Jean, Chermette René. Paris: Lavoisier Tec et Doc, 139-165. ISBN 2-7430-0495-9

Jaenson, TGT, Palsson K, Borg-Karlson, AK. 2006. Evaluation of extracts and oils of mosquito (Diptera: Culicidae) repellent plants from Sweden and Guinea-Bissau. Journal of Medical Entomology, **43**(1): 113-11

Jahandiez, E.& Maire, R., (1932). Catalogue des plantes du Maroc (Spermatophytes et Ptéridophytes). Minerva, Alger. 2 (Dicotyledons Archichlamydae), 489-496.

Kaplan EL and Meier P., 1958. Non parametric estimation from incompJete observations. Journal of the American Statistical Association, Vol. 53, No. 282 (Jun., 1958), pp 457-81.

Keane S., and Ryan MF. 1999: Purification, characterisation, and inhibition by monoterpenes of acetylcholinesterase from the waxmoth, Gallenia mellonella (L.). Insect biochemistry and molecular biology Vol29(12) 1097-1104.

Kerharo, J., Adams, J. G. (1974). La Pharmacopée Sénégalaise Traditionnelle: Plantes Médicinales et Toxiques. In Edition.Vigot Frères,paris (pp. 211-214, 224-225,490).

Khani A, Basavand F and Rakhshani E, 2012. Chemical composition and insecticide activity of lemon verbena essential oil. Journal of Crop Protection ; university of Zabol- Iran ,1(4): 313-320.

Koroghli, K. (2018). Insecticidal activity of rosemary (Rosmarinusofficinalis L.) and peppermint (Menthapiperita L.) essential oils towards adults of the small wheat grain beetleRhyzoperthadominica F.(Coleoptera: Bostrychidae) (Doctoral dissertation, Université Mouloud Mammeri).

Lancien J. 1981. Description of the monoconic trap used for the elimination of tsetse flies in the People's Republic of Congo. Cahiers ORSTOM. Série Entomologie Médicale et Parasitologie, 19:235-238.

Lancien J., 1991. Control of sleeping sickness in south-eastern Uganda by tsetse fly trapping. ORSTOM. Ann. Soc. Belg. Méd. 1991, 71 (Suppl. 1), 35-47.

Laveissière, C., & Couret, D. (1985). Observations on the irritant effect of synthetic pyrethroids on tsetse flies (l). Cahiers d'ORSTOM, Série Entomologie Médicale et Parasitologie, 23, 289-295.

Laveissière C., Couret, D. and Kienon J.P., 1980. Control of riverine tsetse flies using insecticide-impregnated biconical traps in the humid savannah zone. Description of the environment, equipment and method. Cahiers ORSTOM, ser. Ent. méd. et Parasit, 1980. 18 (3), 201- 207.

Laveissière C., Couret D., Manno A. 1987. Importance of the nature of the tissues in tsetse fly trapping. Cahiers ORSTOM. Série Entomologie Médicale et Parasitologie, 25(34): 133-143.

Laveissière C., Grébaut P. 1990. Recherches sur les pièges à glossines (Diptera: Glossinidae): Mise au point d'un modèle économique: Le piège "Vavoua". Tropical Medicine and Parasitology, 41: 185-192.

Leak, S. A., 1999. Tsetse biology and ecology. Their role in the epidemiology and control of trypanosomosis. CABI publishing, UK, 529 pages.

Lenoir L, 2011. Protective effect of fragrant verbena polyphenols in a rat model of colonic inflammation: Université d'Auvergne-Clermont-Ferrand I.

Maillard J. C. and Provost A., 1975. Research into the pathogenic power of Bacillus thuringiensis on tsetse flies (Diptera-Muscidae). Study on Glossina tachinoides in the Republic of Chad. Revue d'Elevage et de Médecine vétérinaire des Pays tropicaux, 1975. 28 (1): 61-65.

Makoundou, P. B., Cuisance, D., Duvallet, G., & Guillet, P. (1995). Laboratory study of the effects of a natural insecticide extracted from neem (Azadirachta indica A. Juss) on Glossina fuscipes Newstead, 1910 (Diptera: Glossinidae). Revue d'élevage et de médecine vétérinaire des pays tropicaux, 48(4), 339-345.

Manal, A.A., Abd El-razik & Gamal, M.M. (2013). Efficacy of some plant products and two conventional insecticides and their residual activities against Callosobrochus maculatus (F.). American Journal of Biochemistry and Molecular **Biology 3(4):** 356-368.

Mawuena K. and Yacnambe S., 1988. L'utilisation des pièges et écrans imprégnés d'insecticide pour la lutte contre la trypanosomose animale. Revue Elev. Méd. vét. Pays trop ..1988,41 (1),93-96.

Mérot P., Politzar H., Tamboura l, and Cuisance D., (1984). Results of a campaign to control riverine tsetse flies in Burkina using deltamethrin-impregnated screens. Revue Elev. Méd. vét. Pays trop, 1984,37 (2), 175-184.

Moloo S. K., 1993. The distribution of Glossina species in Africa and their natural hosts. Insect Science and Its Application, 14 (4): 511-527.

Nacoulma OG, 1996. Medicinal Plants and Their Traditional Uses in Burkina Faso. Ph.D.Thesis. University of Ouagadougou 328.

Nadio, N. A., Poutouli, W. P., Laba, B., Tozoou, P., Bokobana, M. E., Koba, K., ... & Sanda, K. (2016). Insecticidal and repellent properties of Ocimum sanctum L. essential oil towards Dysdercus voelkeri Schmidt (Heteroptera; Pyrrhocoridae). Sciences de la vie, de la terre et agronomie, 3(2).

Ouedraogo, I., Sawadogo, A., Nebie, R. C., & Dakouo, D. (2016). Evaluation of the toxicity of Cymbopogon nardus (L) and Ocimum gratissimum (L) essential oils against Sitophilus zeamais Motsch and Rhyzopertha dominica F, the main insect pests of maize in storage.... International Journal of Biological and Chemical Sciences, 10(2), 695-705.

Parsons, W. T., Cuthbertson, E. G. (1992). Noxious Weeds of Australia. In Data Press,Melbourne/Sydney, 490-492.

Pasma Mache Nkouandou, Patrick Akono Ntonga, Christelle Awansi Djeukam, Pierre Michel Jazet Dongmo, Chantal Menut 2020. Evaluation of the insecticidal properties of essential oils of some Zingiberaceae against Anopheles gambiae s. l. larvae collected in Ayos (southern Cameroon). Journal of Animal & Plant Sciences (J.Anim.Plant Sci. 2020 ISSN 2071-7024) Vol.43 (3): 7469-7482.

Pollock J. N. (Ed.). (1982). Training manual for tsetse control personnel (Vol. 1, p. 274). Rome, Italy: Food and Agriculture Organization of the United Nations.

Pollock J.N., 1996. Ecology and behaviour of tsetse flies. Manual of tsetse fly control volume 2. PAO. Rome (Italy). 117 pages.

Savadogo, S., Sambare, O., Sereme, A., & Thiombiano, A. (2016). Traditional methods of insect and tick control among the Mossé in Burkina Faso. Journal of Applied Biosciences, 105, 10120-10133.

Simo, G., Rayaisse, JB (2015). Challenges to eliminating sleeping sickness in West and Central Africa: sustainable control of animal trypanosomiasis as an indispensable approach to achieve the goal. Parasite Vectors 8, 640 https://doi.org/10.1186/s13071-015-1254-y

Solano, P., Sidibe, I. and Rotureau, B. (2018). Tsetse flies (Diptera: Glossinidae), in D. Fontenille,G. Duvallet and V. Robert, eds, 'Entomologie médicale et vétérinaire', number chap.15, IRD Editions, pp. 367-389.

Somda I., Leth V., and Sérémé P., (2007), Antifungal effect of Cymbopogon citratus, Eucalyptus camaldulensis and Azadirachta indica oil extracts on sorghum seed-borne fungi, Asian Journal of Plant Sciences, 6 (8), 1182-1189.

Swallow, B. 2000. Impacts of Trypanosomiasis on African Agriculture, Food and Agriculture Organization of the United Nations, Rome.

Rajashekar Y; Ravindra KV and Bakthavatsalam N. 2012. Leaves of Lantana camara

Linn. (Verbenaceae) as a potential insecticide for the management of three species of insect pests of stored cereals. J Food Sci Technol, 2491. P.1-6.

Tia, E. V., Cisse, M., Douan, G. B., & Kone, A. (2019). Comparative study of the insecticidal effect of Cymbopogon citratus DC and Ocimum canum Sims essential oils on Cylas puncticollis Boheman, a sweet potato weevil. International Journal of Biological and Chemical Sciences, 13(3), 1789-1799.

Traore N., Sidibe L; Bouare, S 1991. Antimicrobial activities of essential oils of Eucalyptus citriodoraHook and Eucalyptus houseanaW.Fitzg. ex Maiden. Int. J. Biol. Chem. Sci. 7(2): 800-804.

Vale, G.A., Hargrove, J. W., Chamisa, A., Grant, I.F., Torr, S.J., (2015). Pyrethroid Treatment of Cattle for Tsetse Control: Reducing Its Impact on Dung Fauna. PLoS Negl. Trop. Dis. 9.

Vreysen, M. J., Seck, M. T., Sall, B. and Bouyer, J. (2013), 'Tsetse flies: their biology and control using area-wide integrated pest management approaches', Journal of invertebrate pathology **112**, S15-S25. 2, 3, 30, 49, 50.

Yerbanga, RS, Rayaisse, JB., Vantaux, (2016). Neemazal ® as a possible alternative tool for malaria and African trypanosomiasis control? Parasite Vectors 9 , 263 (https://doi.org/10.1186/s13071-016-1538-x

Wangrawa, D. W., Ochomo, E., Upshur, F., Zanre, N., Borovsky, D., Lahondere, C., & Sanon, A. (2022). Essential oils and their binary combinations have synergistic and antagonistic insecticidal properties against Anopheles gambiae sl (Diptera: Culicidae). Biocatalysis and Agricultural Biotechnology, 42, 102347. https://doi.org/10.1016/j.bcab.2022.102347.

Zahran, H. E. D. M., Abou-Taleb, H. K., & Abdelgaleil, S. A. (2017). Adulticidal, larvicidal and biochemical properties of essential oils against Culex pipiens L. Journal of Asia-Pacific Entomology, 20(1), 133-139.

APPENDICES

Appendix 1: Manipulation in the laboratory.

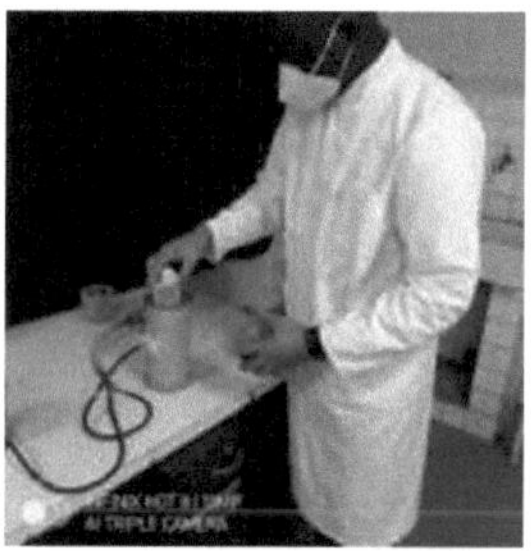

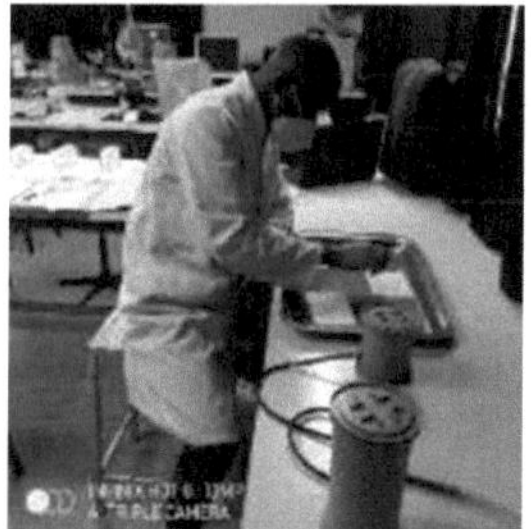

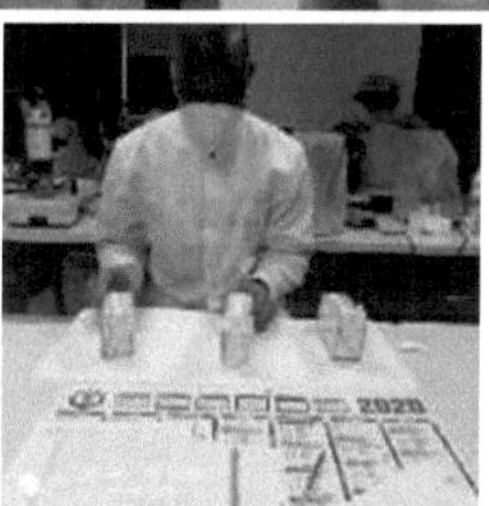

Putting Glossins to sleep with CO2

Tarsal contact of flies

Observation of KD and Mortality.

Appendix 2: Technical equipment.

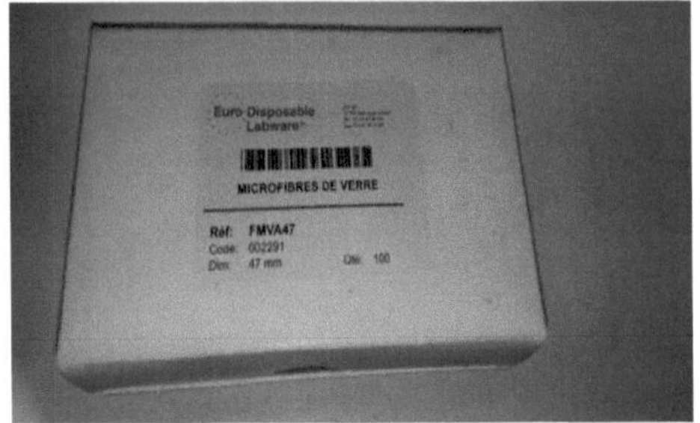

Whatman microfibre paper

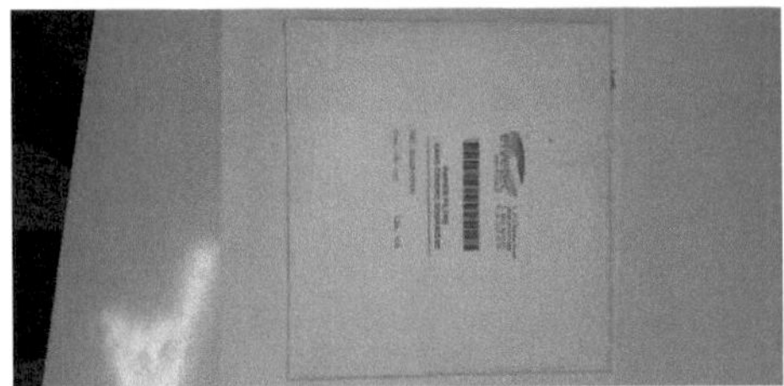

Ashless filter paper degreases

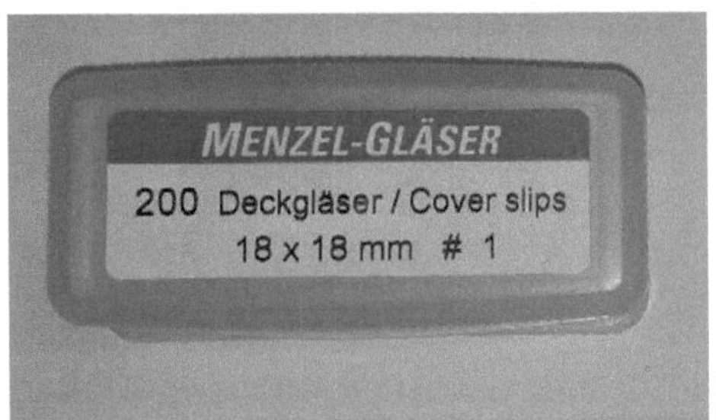

Lamella

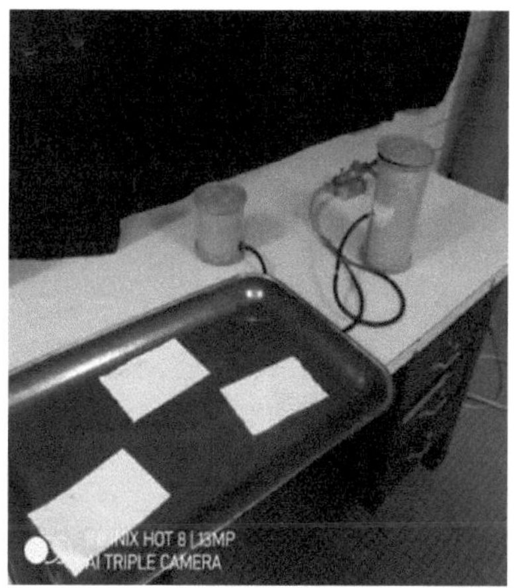

Device for putting tsetse flies to sleep and handling tray

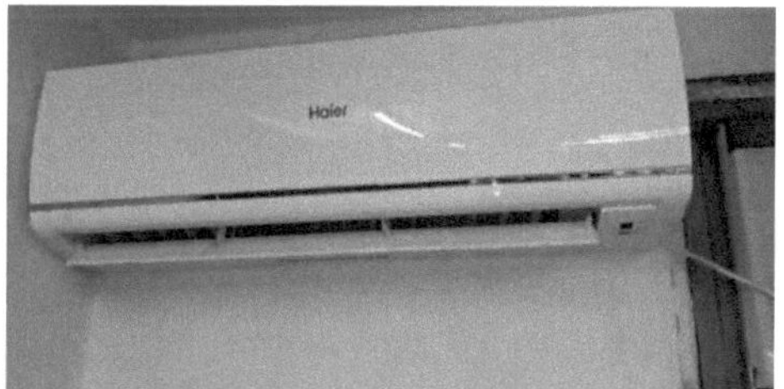

Air conditioning

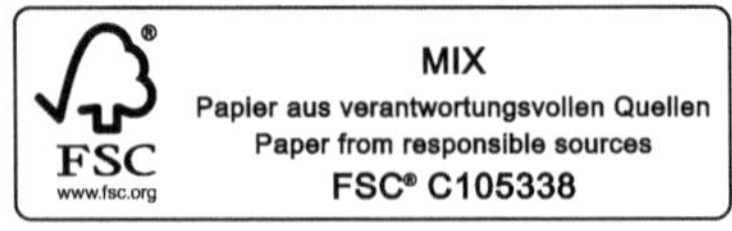

Printed by Books on Demand GmbH, Norderstedt / Germany